I0414922

Design by:

CITY JOURNALS
© 2019

Cover image: © OpenStreetMap contributors

www.ingramcontent.com/pod-product-compliance
Lightning Source LLC
Chambersburg PA
CBHW072055280526
45788CB00006B/2297
9781097997077